Psi-Fit

Developing A Fit Mind

Psi-Fit

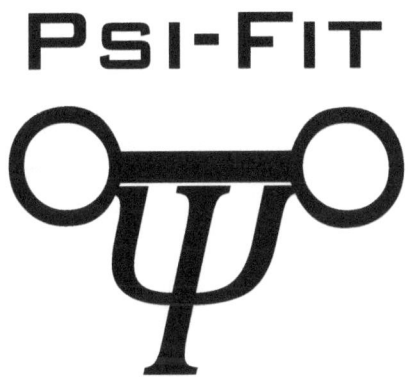

Developing A Fit Mind

Brian Crouse, MA, LIPC
Tiffany Crouse, MAM

This book was created in 2013. Please feel free to share this or make copies. The information is to help others. Do your part and pass it on. Thank you for helping make the world a better place for everyone.

PSI-FIT

Developing A Fit Mind

A New Perspective

Treat people as if they were what
they ought to be and you will
help them become what they
are capable of becoming.

~ Johann Wolfgang Von Goethe

How does one develop A Fit Mind?

For the purpose of this book we will consider fitness the goal we each aspire to. Being able to manage the stress of hectic lives and unforeseen obstacles in a positive manner. Becoming resilient, rebounding back to a feeling of joy, happiness, and fulfilled satisfaction with life.

The general focus of mental health has been on helping people who are suffering, sick, and in despair about their life regain a level of function so they can again contribute to their life and the life of others. We can consider this a return to baseline health or normal function.

Productivity is the goal of business and bosses look at ways to eek out more product for less cost. Managers look for ways to move people to do more with less. They want employees to function well enough to meet the status quo.

Being mentally fit means pushing past baselines. It means aspiring to be above average, to be extraordinary. It means we look to go beyond the status quo.

When we think of a mentally fit person we are looking at those people who seem to always come out smiling. They see opportunities in what others view as obstacles. They lead organizations into the future and make them stronger.

They make a choice to live above the norm.

And there in lies the key.

They make a choice.

They choose to put effort and energy into practicing fitness.

So then the question becomes how do they do this. What do they know that others don't, and can anyone learn to do this?

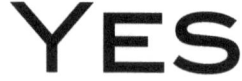

Anyone can learn to be mentally fit. Everyone will start at their own place, and will get as far as they choose to go. There isn't some end goal here, but continued pursuit of excellence, pursuit of fitness.

The only competition is with who you were and your level of function the day before. Each day is a new day and with practice and effort, we can be better.

Continuum of Fitness

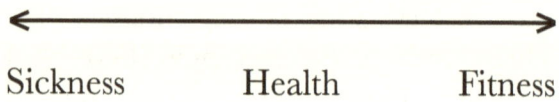

Sickness   Health   Fitness

No matter where you start, you can move toward better fitness.

There are different aspects of Well-being. Each person comes with differing preferences related to these. We may see one as more important or valuable than the others. The person looking to be fit though will work to incorporate each of these into their life.

Along with the Aspects of Well-being, there are Core Functions of mental fitness. Some may be easier than others. Often we have picked up poor habits so need to relearn how to do things. With patience and practice, we find new habits and learn to function better. We can change our reactions and respond better.

Choice is the base for all growth within this process. All the power of mental fitness comes from making a decision, and this is an explosive power that propels us toward our goals and dreams. If we continue to flounder in indecision then we leak power, leaving us drained. By procrastinating we miss opportunities to become fit, to become extraordinary.

Will and Persistence are the vehicles that get us to our destination. By participating in a Mental WOD (Workout of the Day) we become stronger. We improve our ability to make choices and to follow through. Our ability to adapt to change and persevere on the path toward our goals become greater. The interactions we have with others become more meaningful and satisfying.

Aspects of Wellbeing

I have decided to be happy, because it
is good for my health.

~ Voltaire

There are 5 Aspects of Well-being we focus on in pursuit of A Fit Mind.

Security
Freedom
Connection
Worth
Purpose

Each of these is important and interconnected. To be mentally fit, each aspect must be present. While a person can function for a while if one of these is missing or reduced, unless they are able to compensate they will begin to lose fitness and eventually mental health.

Counselors and other mental health professionals are experienced in helping people move from the realms of sickness back to basic health. They remain valuable in our society for this reason, but often the training they have leaves them ill equipped to help people attain mental fitness.

The process of therapy and counseling doesn't have the goal of fitness. The system of compensation is not based on fitness. It is not the current perspective of mental health services to get people beyond baseline function.

Life Coaches work with those who are functioning in a decent manner and help them focus their energy and effort to improve in different parts of their life. They help people move beyond baseline function and toward the idea of fitness, but generally only in certain areas.

These professionals and others can be helpful guides on the way to having A Fit Mind, but it comes down to the individual wanting it bad enough to put in the effort and time.

This book is only another guide.

A model for achievement.

It is the adoption of a new lifestyle and new perspective which moves us toward optimal mental fitness.

Security

The reason we struggle with insecurity
is because we compare our behind-
the-scenes with everyone else's
highlight reel.

~ Steve Furtick

The aspect of Security includes the basic needs of shelter, food, water, and anything else that keeps a body going. These needs are those that if a person goes without for a short period of time, their physiological health decreases significantly.

Another part of Security is feeling and being safe. This is a matter for the person to decide, but if we remain in heightened states of alertness for danger, it takes away from our ability to see anything else. If we can work to engineer a safe environment, then we can go about the business of developing A Fit Mind.

Without proper nutrition, a person isn't able to think, act, or choose as effectively. This isn't a book about what is and is not healthy to eat. For this purpose, let's settle with eating foods that make you feel better, and provide you with the sustenance to focus on making better choices.

Physical exercise has many benefits for people, and lives have become more sedentary with the modernization of society. Again, the purposes of this guide is not to promote a specific exercise, but rather to promote the person finding some form of exercise to improve their overall health. It could be as simple as taking the first open parking stall rather than seeking out one closer to the store.

The point is that if the basic needs and sense of safety are not met then a person will struggle to maintain their Well-Being. If we can adequately meet our survival needs then we can begin to move toward thriving.

Freedom

I am not what happened to me.
I am what I choose to become.

~ Carl Gustav Jung

The aspect of Freedom relates to a person's ability to make decisions. We have a higher sense of Well-Being when we have input into the course of our lives.

When oppressed or coerced into actions counter to our desire we lose our sense of control. When this happens we can take desperate measures to get back control, often harming our relationships.

When we exercise our freedom, we advocate for ourselves. We find our voice and we begin to speak up for what we want, for what we believe in. We choose to stand up for our values and to better represent our status.

To promote our sense of Freedom requires us to seek our power regardless of the situation. We need to explore our options and identify the opportunities for forward movement.

This can be a struggle at times, but with practice we become better at identifying the different choices available and making decisions that benefit our journey toward better Well-Being.

Connection

Associate yourself with people
of good quality.

~ Booker T. Washington

We are each in a relationship with the people around us. We are connected in an expansive web to others. The aspect of Connection focuses on our sense of belonging and inclusion within the network of our relationships.

Our interactions with others either strengthens or weakens our sense of Connection. Our Well-Being improves when we make choices to strengthen our relationships.

We can do this by demonstrating empathy, and we all have the skills to nurture others. We are social creatures by nature and gain strength to be better through our connections.

We choose how much we let the affairs of others affect us and we choose our level of response. We can decide whether we act with kindness to others.

Damage is done in our relationships by taking information others give personally. If we can recognize it as their best effort to communicate their current struggle and need for support, then we can respond with compassion.

Worth

Everybody is a genius, but if you judge
a fish by its ability to climb a tree,
it will live its whole life
believing that it is stupid.

~ Albert Einstein.

What is the true value of a person? Many people are given the idea they only have Worth if they do as someone with more power or authority says.

This leads to the false belief that our Worth is tied to the opinions of others and so our Well-Being is placed on a roller-coaster ride that often ends in despair, because others are practiced at pointing out our faults.

It is equally unhealthy to tie our Worth to the praise we get for actions. It reinforces the same concept that the thoughts of others determines our value. Praise is like candy, gobble up too much of it and it will make you sick.

In the premise of A Fit Mind, Worth is not tied to the opinions of others, or even our opinion of ourselves. Our Worth is intrinsic, and not subject to the vacillations of judgment.

Worth is our source of power, our ability to impact the world. It is the identity and knowledge of who we are at our core. Our values and confidence in who we are, and the importance we have in the world. These are the concepts of Worth.

Our Well-Being is increased by choosing activities and thoughts that give us the confidence to make the best decisions for our lives, outside of the opinions of others.

Purpose

When I do good, I feel good.
When I do bad, I feel bad.
That's my religion.

~ Abraham Lincoln

We all move toward building meaning into our lives. Purpose focuses on what makes our existence important.

Our passions are what clue us in to our Purpose. When we are engaged in a passionate pursuit we experience a bend in the way we experience time. This is commonly known as flow, and people experience it when they are living out their purpose.

Time becomes twisted and hours fly by. We look up from a project and darkness has fallen, or the sun is coming up again.

Our inner critic, the part of us that judges what we do, shuts down. We are in the zone, and in this mental space we create new realities.

This is the place where activity becomes play. We have fun without effort. We reach our bliss. As we develop A Fit Mind, we more easily attain this experience. We begin to have more time spent in play and less in work.

We shape our lives around flow, play, fun, and bliss. We shape our lives around passion. We live out our Purpose.

Core Functions

Instead of wondering when your next vacation is, maybe you should set up a life you don't need to escape from.

~ Seth Godin

There are 5 Core Functions
of A Fit Mind.

Do It Now
Habitual Excellence
Focal Shift
Conserving Resources
Pulling Strings

By way of these functions, we are able to improve the Aspects of Well-being. We can improve the function of these and the way we interact in the world. Through practice and discipline we can shape our mind to excel regardless of the situation.

We learn to make better decisions and to do actions faster. We are able to endure more stress for greater periods of time because we are mentally fit. There is also a quicker rebound back to fitness even if we experience catastrophic events.

Being mentally fit prepares us to be of greater service to others and to be less traumatized by negative outcomes. We are able to make more significant impacts on our communities and realize greater success in all our endeavors.

We are better managers, better employees, and better co-workers. We become leaders in our organizations and communities.

We become more aware of our connections and our influence in the world. We recognize the power we have over our lives and what it means to experience optimal mental function.

People with A Fit Mind see opportunities in their life and experience a greater sense of meaning in their activities whether it be work, play, relaxing, spending time with family, or another pursuit they choose.

Do It Now

If we wait until we're ready we'll be
waiting for the rest of our lives.

~ Lemony Snicket

Each time we encounter a task we have the option to either do it or put it off. By putting things off in a consistent manner we create traps. These traps limit our potential for spontaneity, fun, happiness, and satisfaction.

We procrastinate and eliminate our freedom, shackling ourselves to deadlines, killing ourselves with obligations. The key to the freedom we seek is by embracing the idea of Do It Now.

There is no moment but now. Now is unfolding into the future and it will do so in the direction of our choice. Will we move forward or will we try to remain where we are?

We use our imagination to envision a future, and it is our essential task to move the present, the now, toward that future. Why wait to get to the future you want.

What are you waiting for?

When we Do It Now:

We can provide for our basic needs and assure our Security.

We create a pattern that gives us back our Freedom.

Our relationships are happening now. Now is the only time we can have a Connection with others.

We express our Worth by stepping forward, not by holding back and waiting.

Our Purpose, our passion, our ability to enter a flow state will never happen if our choice is to procrastinate.

So go out there and

Do Something

Do It Now

Habitual Excellence

The only limits you have are
the limits you believe.

~ Wayne Dyer

When we practice we become better. The heart of Habitual Excellence is to practice until we are better. What happens though is there is always a new mark to aim for.

This may seem daunting. We are so used to having goals with a specific end-point. Better is not a specific end point. It is a shifting end-point.

There is no competition with Habitual Excellence. We are only measured by who we were, what we did, and how we acted the year, week, day, second before as compared to who we are becoming.

We get to try again, always.

The start-point is as shifting as the end-point. We practice Excellence until the practice is Habit. It becomes painful to not push, to not pursue better.

If we create Habitual Excellence:

We find better, more satisfying ways of providing for our Security.

Our sense of Freedom is enhanced by the better choices we make.

We seek out ways to build stronger, more beneficial Connections with others.

Our movement toward better lets us see and display our Worth.

The internal editor is silenced by shifting start-points and end-points, freeing us to live our Purpose.

Focal Shift

Sometimes it's to your advantage for
people to think you're crazy.

~ Thelonious Monk

What we expect to see is what we end up seeing. We believe we are focused and paying attention to what we need to so we can succeed.

And we look at the wrong things. We want to be successful but we identify our failures.

Why put a spotlight on mistakes?

What we focus on tends to happen. What we look for we find. If we look for problems then we will find them, in abundance. When we seek mistakes we make mistakes.

Our attention is limited.

We can only focus on one thing at a time.

Opportunity is the flip side of obstacle.

Our world is created by what we focus on, what we pay attention to. If we choose to experience a Focal Shift, we choose to create a different reality.

If we focus on success we experience success. The more we look for what is right the more we see what is right in the world. The more we focus on the positive, the fewer negatives we see.

By choosing to make a Focal Shift:

We see how our needs are already met. We open ourselves up to the Security we possess.

We see options and have the Freedom to choose our path to the future.

Our Connection is improved because we see what is good and kind about others.

We celebrate our Worth and the Worth of others, and focus our power on possibility.

Our Purpose gains focus. We notice and can enhance the fun and joy in the world.

Conserving Resources

Make it simple, but significant.

~ Don Draper

We can be conservationists of any resource. We have the power to redefine what is of use to us in our lives. When we work to Conserve Resources we seek ways to be more efficient.

We also look at how quality is of greater value than quantity. Having more doesn't mean we have a better life. It doesn't mean we are better at meeting our needs. We work to preserve and improve what we already have, whether it be a possession or a relationship.

Being a conservationist means we find better ways to use what is available. We become grateful for what we have and creative in how to use it. We find inspiration in simplicity.

We find ways to simplify, to make things elegant, and to serve multiple uses.

We conserve our energy by taking fewer steps. We reduce the superfluous and seek the core, the meaning, the heart of material and being.

Through the practice of Conserving Resources:

We find Security by using the available resources in a more elegant manner.

We foster our Freedom by engaging our creativity and power of choice.

Our Connection to people improves exponentially as we focus on quality.

Our Worth is more fully realized by reducing the leakage of our power.

We find Purpose when distractions are reduced. Our meaning is amplified.

Uncomplicate Your Life.

Spend your resources making
the world a better place.

Live Fulfilled

Pulling Strings

Our lives are defined by opportunities,
even the ones we miss.

~ F. Scott Fitzgerald

Will you be the one Pulling Strings or will you be the puppet of a mad marionette?

We all feel pulled around at times, like someone else is in charge of what is happening. This usually happens when we are trying to work against the flow of life. We get caught up in the maelstrom of life and get battered and bruised.

Pulling Strings is stepping back, finding a way to be calm. When we find our center and our personal peace it is like we enter the eye of the storm. Everything spins around us but we can see the best path forward.

When we are Pulling Strings we can leverage the opportunities others miss. We can capitalize on our strengths, our skills, and our talents. We can experience all the benefits of A Fit Mind.

When we are being our true, authentic self then we are in charge of our life. We can pull the strings of the universe and position ourselves to be exceptional. We can be in the right place at the right time more often, because we choose the times and places.

We no longer must wait for opportunity
to strike.

We create the opportunity.

As we start Pulling Strings:

We feel less threatened by the chaos of the world and recognize our Security despite circumstances.

We experience Freedom from obligation and instead choose the best option.

We find a stronger Connection in the web of our network and can reap the benefits.

We help others to see their Worth and recognize their potential.

We begin to see how our Purpose is intertwined with everyone else's.

Exercising Choice

Whatever the present moment
contains, embrace it as if
you had chose it.

~ Eckhardt Tolle

Decision is the power that drives our lives.

Will keeps us on track toward our desires, returning to the course despite detours.

Persistence is the belief dreams will come true if we keep moving forward.

The process of Exercising Choice strengthens our confidence to make a decision, trains our will to stay true, and bolsters our persistence to keep making the attempt.

The process is simple.

With regard to the Aspects of Well-Being and by utilizing the Core Functions we develop…

A Fit Mind.

The Threshold Game:

Think for a moment how many doors you pass through each day.

A lot right?

To make something become a habit we have to do, or think, it over and over. What happens if we can use a simple cue to practice a mental exercise? What if we select a cue that happens multiple times a day?

We could start to develop A Fit Mind.

Given a week of practice, using a door as a cue, we can engrain an new way of thinking.

Given a month of practice we gain a new approach to the world.

Given a year of practice we can gain a new perspective.

Imagine who you could be one year from now.

How much more free you could be.

How much better your relationships could be.

How much more meaning your life could have.

Imagine that and then let's start the process of moving the present toward that future.

Following are 52 choices. One for each week. These are only a guide and can be done in any order. And please exchange any of them for ones that match your personal goals better.

I choose to have fun.

I choose to be curious.

I choose to be polite.

I choose to be calm.

I choose to try.

I choose to forgive.

I choose to be grateful.

I choose to act with grace.

I choose to adapt.

I choose to be creative.

I choose to act with compassion.

I choose to be responsible.

I choose to listen.

I choose to smile.

I choose to be helpful.

I choose to advocate for others.

I choose to act with courage.

I choose to be kind.

I choose to be enthusiastic.

I choose to be authentic.

I choose to be humble.

I choose to be optimistic.

I choose to be playful.

I choose to reach out to others.

I choose to demonstrate self-control.

I choose to be prudent.

I choose to take risks.

I choose to be imaginative.

I choose to act with patience.

I choose to learn.

I choose to let go.

I choose to find opportunity.

I choose to be active.

I choose to celebrate what's right.

I choose to act with confidence.

I choose to be generous.

I choose to daydream.

I choose to commit.

I choose to be passionate.

I choose to serve.

I choose to be tranquil.

I choose to lead.

I choose to act with intention.

I choose to collaborate.

I choose to seek moments of awe.

I choose to teach.

I choose to endure.

I choose to be fair.

I choose to be empathetic.

I choose to be spontaneous.

I choose to act better.

I choose to be attentive.

Mental WODs

You must learn a new way to think
before you can master
a new way to be.

~ Marianne Williamson

WOD is WorkOut of the Day. These are brief activities that take up to 5—10 minutes to complete. Stack them up for a longer workout. It is amazing what can happen by spending 10—20 minutes a day Working Out your Mind.

Start by choosing one of the following experiences for your WOD. Some are easier than others and some may be quite a challenge depending on your current strengths and level of comfort. There is no wrong way to do these. It is about making the choice and putting in the effort.

As you begin to get more comfortable, add more experiences to your WOD. This isn't to be intrusive in your life, but it does need to challenge you and push some boundaries. It is outside of our comfort zone where we begin to change.

Please enjoy, and add to the list with your own challenges. Please share these with us and we will compile a list of WOD experiences. It is our hope to incorporate technology into the Psi-Fit adventure and have an active web presence and make use of apps on smart devices.

Take a brisk walk, or exercise, for 5 minutes

Write out 5 things that went right in the past 24 hours.

Write a letter to someone.

Compliment the first 5 people you meet today.

Hold the door open for others today.

Turn off your electronics for 5 minutes and just sit.

Take 25 deep breaths. Count to two on inhale. Hold for two. Exhale for two. Repeat.

Write out 5 things you're grateful for.

Whistle on your way to places.

Listen to NPR for 10 minutes.

Find 5 inspiring quotes.

Write a thank you note to someone and deliver it.

Pay for someone's lunch.

Commit 5 Acts of Kindness.

Think about a T-Rex making a bed, doing a pull up, tying a tie, putting on a bowler hat.

Play tag with someone.

Have a conversation with a child.

Eat something amazing and savor the taste.

For today, use the opposite of your preferred hand to eat, brush your teeth, write.

Learn a new joke and tell it to someone.

Read a short story in a genre you don't like.

Sit on the floor and look around the room you're in.

Ask someone how they are and don't settle for a one word answer.

Play the angel's advocate.

Make three conversations be all about the other person.

Say "yes" to any reasonable request.

Imagine you're a superhero in disguise.

Switch absolute language (should, have to, must) to preference language (could, get to, can).

Tell someone why you love them.

Eat dessert first.

Listen to a different radio station or different genre of music for the day.

Say sir and ma'am to everyone for a day.

Say thank you when leaving a room.

Practice your handshake.

Spend your latte money on a gift for someone.

Ask 3 people if they would like a hug.

Roll down the windows and blare your music.

For a day, only answer direct questions and make your answers brief.

Pay someone a dollar for being them.

Write a poem.

Drink a glass of water and savor the sensation.

Pick a word, look it up in a thesaurus and then use one of the synonyms.

Look at a piece of art and imagine painting, drawing, sculpting, creating it.

Dance, spin, rock, just move in a different way.

Tell people they are amazing.

Think about someone who you are happy with.

Remember the best vacation you have ever been on.

Play a new game.

Pretend the power went out for an evening.

Eat a piece of chocolate.

Take a different route to a routine destination.

Chew a piece of bubble gum.

Write out 5 things that will go right in the next 24 hours.

Start something new.

Share a secret.

Stand up for someone else.

Race someone.

Imitate your favorite animal for 5 minutes.

Hold your breath for as long as possible.

Laugh.

Put a puzzle together except the last piece and leave it for someone else to finish.

Spend 10 minutes in a park or garden or anywhere else there are numerous plants.

Open up a book and count the words on the page.

Build something out of blocks.

Ask someone to help you with something.

Let go of a grudge.

Choose a motto of the day.

See the good in someone you struggle to get along with.

Watch the second hand go by on a clock for twice the number of seconds of your age.

Carry a pen or pencil with you and take notes about the beauty you see.

Sign your name like you're a famous artist for the day.

Learn a magic trick.

Do a crossword.

Change some part of your outfit at lunch and see who notices.

Play the quiet game. You can either have others join or just do it on your own.

Imagine the life story of someone you see on the street or in front of you in line. Get detailed.

Learn how to say something in a different language.

Speak in third person for as long as you can.

Name 1 gratitude for each letter of the alphabet.

Complete a sudoko or logic puzzle.

Rearrange some furniture in your office or home.

Cook something new.

Call someone you consider a mentor and tell them thank you.

Reflect on the most meaningful event of the past week.

Dress up more than normal today.

Wrap up in a warm-from-the-dryer blanket.

Sit outside for five minutes.

Count squirrels or birds or some other plentiful animal on your next trip out of the house.

Get lost and take your time finding your way back.

Try to talk with or without your hands, whichever is the opposite of your norm.

Do something courageous.

Imagine what you would do if money were no object.

Declutter your workspace or livespace.

Identify 5 time-sucks and pick one to stop doing for the day.

Trust someone to take care of something.

Play spin-doctor. Reframe statements to the positive.

Act like a REF - Respect, Empathy, Fairness.

Make something out of play-dough.

Become enthused about the mundane.

Practice a skill or talent for 10 minutes.

Author Info

Brian is a Mental Health Counselor with over a decade of experience in helping people find better ways to manage their lives. He has become more convinced the current system is not good enough to have people live full lives. This pushed him to examine what makes people excel in life and share the information.

Tiffany uses her skills as a life coach to enhance the growth of others toward their potential. She studied Leadership and Management and has extensive experience working in non-profit organizations. She continues to find ways to leverage the passions of others to improve communities and help people live more fulfilled lives.

Please check out our FaceBook page at:
http://bit.ly/Psi-Fit
for more information and share stories
about your Psi-Fit adventure.